I'm Katie's Mom

I'm Katie's Mom

Pointers for Professionals
and Parents of the Disabled

Barbara B. Holdcroft, Ph.D.

VANTAGE PRESS
New York

The opinions expressed herein are solely those of the author. Readers should seek the advice of their personal physician and/or therapist before embarking on any new medical or therapeutic program.

FIRST EDITION

Published by Vantage Press, Inc.
419 Park Ave. South, New York, NY 10016

Manufactured in the United States of America
ISBN: 978-0-533-15789-1

Library of Congress Catalog Card No.: 2007902934

0 9 8 7 6 5 4 3 2 1

To Katie, the catalyst for my learning and much growth in our family. Special thanks to Maryjane Heagney for her inspiration and to Mary Virginia Gray for editorial direction.

Contents

Introduction

Hi, I'm Katie's Mom. Often that is my only identity. That's the one that is important to Katie, my daughter with a disability. It is certainly the only identity that counts within her circle. My name is totally unimportant.

If you are reading this, you most likely have a child who has been diagnosed with a disability, or perhaps you are a professional who assists in the education and care of those with a disability. Contrary to the misconceptions of conventional society, dealing with those who are physically and mentally challenged is not always sad and depressing or a negative experience. This can be a very positive experience and an individual challenge to become more than you thought you could be. There are a great many resources available and parenting this child, or choice of your career in this field, can become the most positive force in your life.

I am writing this because pertinent advice and information regarding raising a child with a disability is often difficult to obtain, especially from parents who "have been there." In my experience, it took several years to find out how to help myself, my daughter, our family, and about the available agencies and services. Additionally, the scope and number of services has dramatically increased, at least in my geographic area, in the twenty-six years of parenting Katie. I hope that this might be a guide for some parents, and perhaps those in the field who are the professionals and caregivers.

Being a parent of a "normal" child is no "cake-walk" if

you take your responsibility seriously. Parents often disagree regarding the best parenting style, there are miscommunications, and differences of opinion. Sometimes arguments and even divorce occur.

There are a great many similarities between caring for a "normal" child and caring for a child with a disability. Many of the same issues arise, and these difficulties are often magnified with parenting of a child with disabilities. Therefore, I think that advice is sorely needed, and too often, not forthcoming.

As with normal children, one of the caregivers becomes the "primary caregiver." Over time, and as the child ages, the primary caregiver may change. It has been a little different in my household. Katie has identified most closely with me, but this has not changed with age. Although she enjoys the company of her dad and her brother, she still relies on me.

My daughter has been diagnosed as being "multihandicapped" indicating that a number of disabilities challenge her. The most glaring is her inability to speak, to form words. Katie can make sounds, and her receptive language is very good. This means that she can truly understand and comprehend most of what is said in conversation, but is unable to respond verbally. This is a factor in her being able to learn. Her disabilities include motor control issues, especially small motor activities. It is very difficult for her to hold a pen or pencil correctly to write, or even to color with broad strokes. Further, psychological tests indicate that on some cognitive level, that is difficult to determine, there are deficiencies. This means that things like time and other abstract concepts pose a problem for Katie.

Regardless, these disabilities are not as severe as some others. For that we are most grateful. It also has given us the opportunity to "forge ahead" and challenge Katie on many fronts that might be inaccessible for many others with different forms of a disability.

Additionally, we have been very blessed on two other fronts: Katie has never been unhealthy or medically challenged, and she has a permanently cheerful temperament. There has never been any ongoing life-threatening medical condition that required extended hospitalization. And the perpetually happy disposition and enthusiasm Katie brings to her everyday life is infectious. Her own optimism and affection have gone a long way in boosting my confidence and providing strength to move on. These two factors permeate the experiences and information found in these pages.

The ideas and stories in this book relate to the experiences within the context of my particular family. It is a description of dealing with Katie and her limitations on a daily basis over her lifetime.

There is the disappointment of realizing she may never go to college, get married, and produce cuddly grandchildren. There have certainly been moments of distress and concern in contemplating the "what next" of this story. But there are other dreams and goals that can be achieved if one is not complacent and the challenge is embraced.

Because Katie is unable to verbally express her thoughts, yet I can easily observe her features and actions, I have taken an unusual approach to writing. Each chapter will begin with my own experience on a particular topic, and then I will often add what I imagine to be Katie's thoughts on the experience. Even though Katie has disabilities, I see her as an individual with emotions and thoughts of her own. They cannot be dismissed, and I will attempt to "verbalize" what she cannot. There are many days I surely wish she could express herself.

Finally, a word about myself. Those who know me well cannot fail to observe my own generally positive attitude. As I hope to convey in the following pages, this is not a case of naïve optimism, but rather a hopeful realism. I do not believe that there is some "magic" solution that will make everything "right" and then life will be "normal." Challenges abound on a daily basis, and life can, and does, become frustrating at times. But I believe my attitude is generated by a faith conviction that is balanced by what is actually possible to accomplish in the real world. This is an attitude that has come to me gradually, through numerous difficult days and nights, over twenty-six plus years. I encourage all my readers to develop and cultivate a hopeful realism.

This book will not give all the answers for every situation. It does not and cannot address every conceivable situation. But I hope that it offers some insight into this particular challenge. It will simply detail some of what I have learned in twenty-six years of being "Katie's Mom."

I'm Katie's Mom

One

Diagnosis and Direction

Katie is my second child. Her brother Kent is three-and-a-half years older and "normal" in the medical sense. Both were happy babies. Katie ate well, slept well, and was perpetually pleasant. But before Katie was one year old, my husband and I noticed some delays in her physical development. She was not crawling at an appropriate age which also meant she wasn't trying to walk either.

We lived in New Hampshire for most of Katie's first year. The pediatrician there did not think that these delays were an issue for her age. We felt differently. We took Katie to a neurologist, who did a number of tests. He thought she was still within "normal" limits and told us not to worry yet. A follow-up appointment within six months was suggested.

At about this time my husband was transferred back to Ohio. After the last evaluation, some six to eight months passed without much progress. Katie was now nearly eighteen months old. It was time to seek help again.

After the move, we reconnected with our former family physician. I was blessed to have the services of this great pediatrician. He recognized some lingering developmental delays and was not afraid to suggest further medical evaluation.

An appointment with a second local neurologist was made. This second neurologist went 180 degrees in the other direction from the first neurologist in New Hampshire. He

1

stated that Katie would never be able to function, never be able to feed herself, walk, bathe, or perform any activities of daily living. Institutionalization was recommended. All of this without a diagnosis of her disability!

When I pressed him for a reason, he quite boldly asserted that her head was too small. He proclaimed that her brain and skull had just stopped growing, setting her developmental status at a near-vegetative level.

I was incensed that this was his only diagnosis after four to five hours of examination. Although this was a possible explanation, for me it raised questions. A small head size ran in my family. I knew this. Upon prior examinations my mother, my son, and I all were found to have a small head size. I pressed the doctor to establish "how small was too small" and then had him measure our heads. Guess what? According to that medical analysis, everyone in my immediate family should have received a similar diagnosis of mental disability. Since I possessed both a Bachelor of Education and Masters of Science in Education, it should be apparent why this diagnosis did not satisfy me.

Returning to my trusty pediatrician, I followed his advice to see yet a third neurologist at a local teaching hospital for another diagnosis. Although many tests were conducted over several visits, no clear diagnosis emerged. We even tested for some syndromes that we had seen on television. There appeared to be nothing genetically deficient, and no label for the developmental problems emerged. This was both good and bad.

The good news was that no fatal disease was identified that would take my smiling child from me. The bad news was that no name could be ascribed to Katie's developmental delays, thus depriving us of valuable information and treatments. There was no prognosis to indicate what she was or was not capable of accomplishing in her life. But at least it was established that head size was not to blame for Katie's inability to crawl, walk, or speak on a normal timetable. Although extensive family testing was not available for us at this time, medical advances have made new tests available to diagnose family genetic predispositions.

My work had just begun. I now knew what Katie was not doing. It was time to find out what she could do. This meant more medical tests that focused on defining her abilities not her deficiencies.

We checked her hearing; we tested her inner ear and her balance. And we checked everything that could be checked. I would love to be able to outline all the tests that were performed, but I was not present for a lot of them. At the time, it was the custom to sit in a waiting room while the procedures took place and to receive a verbal report later, hopefully with recommendations. Today a caregiver has more opportunity to observe testing procedures. If being present could upset the outcome, then I certainly would suggest getting a written report naming the specific test, outlining the methods used, listing the outcomes, and interpreting the results. Having this information not only can prevent repeat testing but will aid your memory as time passes.

Armed with all the information from the various doctors and tests, the interventions began. Know that interventions can often begin at the same time testing is done. Katie attended several sessions with developmental psychologists at local hospitals and with agencies that offered treatments. Some suggestions involved working with her balance, and exercise programs were attempted and carried out for many weeks. Katie was enrolled in a variety of "speech classes" in an attempt to coax her to speak. Most courses or therapies lasted from six to eight weeks.

We tried whatever seemed necessary; we tried whatever was available. We tried a number of what seemed to be ineffective interventions. Ultimately, we have no way of knowing if any of these actually helped.

As time passed (twenty-six years to be exact), Katie has learned to walk, run, feed and bathe herself, and perform other household tasks. Why has she been able to accomplish these things? No one really knows, but I have my thoughts.

Katie is a member of our family and has always been treated as an active participant. We virtually took her everywhere even to all her brother's athletic events. She was given the chance to see what "normal" activity was. I truly think she really wanted to be a part of what was going on around her. This became her motivation to learn, and my family and I gave her every opportunity.

Her skills continue to evolve, and we continue to "stretch" her abilities. We set expectations and have been firm about her learning skills, from how to put on Velcro tennis shoes to brushing her teeth to developing her athletic skills.

Although Katie has made great strides in her development, she is still unable to speak words. Her lack of ability to communicate remains the single most obvious delay. There is still no concrete medical reason for this, although there is a suspicion.

In the first trimester of my pregnancy, I developed ventricular tachycardia—my heart beat very fast and very inefficiently. The suspicion is that because of this heart irregularity the speech portion of Katie's brain was denied oxygen while it was developing causing the inability to speak along with some of her other developmental delays. This can't be proven, but it is probably the cause.

A diagosis can be important in treatment for the child or in future family planning or to future generations, but the fact is one may never be found. We will probably never really know, but that has not prevented us from moving on to deal with what each day-to-day situation provides.

The progression from medical opinion to testing to intervention cannot be avoided. Gathering information from many sources, especially many physicians, is crucial to the decisions that need to be made throughout the life of your child. I cannot stress enough the importance of getting a second medical opinion! You will value the professional advice of your pediatrician or your obstetrician or family doctor. The expression "two heads are better than one" also applies to physicians, neurologists, and clinicians. Plural. Many of them. Never be afraid to ask for help.

*   *   *

Hi! My name is Katie. I am a special child with a disability, and there are some things that I cannot do. I cannot talk or write. But there are lots of things that I CAN do. I can swim, ride a bike, go skiing, and go just about everywhere. What I do best is have fun.

I am a lucky girl and have lots of fun things to do every day. But sometimes I get hurt while I am having fun. That is when I have to get help from a doctor. If I am in a hurry to get help, I go to the Emergency Room at a hospital.

I have very weak ankles. I have sprained them several times. When I do this and it hurts badly, my Mom will take me to the Emergency Room. Dad stays home with my brother and the dogs.

When we get to the Emergency Room, I usually ride through the doors in a wheelchair. It is hard to get out of the car but easy to sit in the wheelchair. A nurse comes to check on me. Sometimes I am still crying.

I sit with my Mom while the nurse admits me and puts all my information on the computer. Sometimes I get a little name bracelet to wear while I am there. This also upsets me since I do not like to wear any bracelets or things on my arms.

Eventually I get taken back to a large room where a doctor will see me. Sometimes the nurse will take my temperature and blood pressure while we are there.

The doctor will examine my injury and see how serious it might be. Sometimes I need an x-ray to be taken. I get wheeled to another part of the hospital for this.

In the x-ray room, a special technician will help me to sit on the x-ray table. The x-ray takes a picture of my bones to make sure that none of them are broken. The x-ray does not hurt at all.

After the doctor has had a chance to look at the x-rays, he will come and talk with me and my Mom. The doctor will tell us what is wrong and what to do to make it better. Sometimes there is special medicine to take or a special wrap to wear on my ankles.

After this, we can go home. The nurses usually help me to get back into the car.

Going to the Emergency Room is not always fun, but it is good to know that there is a place to go that can help me get better when I do get hurt.

Two
Attitude Adjustment

Okay, so your child has been diagnosed with mental retardation or developmental delays or other disabilities. Your emotions are colliding. The joy and love you feel for your child has been tempered with fear and uncertainty for the future. Your life just turned upside down. This is not the end of the world. Much can be done.

With your world spinning out of control, where do you begin? Start with attitudes and realize that yours is really the only one that counts; other positive attitudes are added bonuses.

Take a look at yourself and your own attitudes. Examine your own preconceptions regarding those with a disability and the prejudices that may be lurking in your subconscious. Get in touch with your emotions; and discuss them with a trusted friend or with your doctor. Come to grips with the concept of being the parent of a child with disabilities. You love your child, talking or not, walking or not. Let that love guide your actions. You may just find that your world is starting to spin a little slower.

Once you figure out your place in the world and in your child's world, go educate yourself. Find out as much as you can about the disability. Go online. Get a case worker. Contact your local board of mental retardation. Join a parents' support group. Talk with people. Get advice from your doctor.

Since you are with your child probably more than anyone else, make that time count. Talk with your child, even if your child cannot respond. Make observations on the weather, your schedule, the laundry, whatever. Develop a friendship with your child. Communication shows that you care. Spend time with your child. Take a nap together. Watch a video together. Look at your picture albums together.

Now that you have taken control of yourself and that world seems to be falling into a smooth rhythm, take a moment to consider all of the people affected by this situation. The first list is easy—your child, you, your spouse, and your other children. Next think about extended family—grandparents, aunts, uncles, cousins, nieces, nephews, step relations, and others. Think a little harder about the next list. Include close friends, neighbors, parishioners, tennis buddies, club members, colleagues. Now stretch just a little farther and think about the bank teller, the cashier at your favorite supermarket, the pharmacist, your attorney, the handyman, and all the others your life touches occasionally. All of these people will have thoughts, feelings, and opinions about your child. Many of these will be preconceived opinions. Many people will form opinions through ignorance and lack of experience. You have the ability to help change or mold many of their ideas.

The process of changing the attitudes of others is much the same as dealing with your own attitudes. Become visible in the community. If possible, take your child with you on errands, to shop, to church, to your other children's activities. Take a walk around the neighborhood. Engage your child in the activities of siblings and relatives. This allows people to confront their own attitudes. Give people the opportunity to interact with your child and get to know her as a real person, not a medical condition.

You took the time to educate yourself; now educate your

family, friends, and neighbors. By developing your own expertise, you can now give that knowledge to everyone who interacts with your child. Help dispel whatever myths and falsehoods that may exist. This is often the most difficult task.

Never rely just on words. Know that the example you set is the greatest educational tool there is. How you treat your child will show others how to respond to her.

By changing attitudes you gain some control over that ever revolving world. Your child will benefit from all the stimulation. You will benefit by not only having a companion to share your day with but by creating a bond that will last a lifetime.

If you are paying attention, all of this will cause you to re-evaluate the priorities in your life. That was probably the single-most valuable lesson for me. Before Katie, I scheduled myself tightly, by the hour, perhaps counting my worth by what I was able to accomplish in one day. It took a while—a year or so—but eventually I realized my own priorities needed re-evaluation. This was both a painful and yet eye-opening experience for me. All my daily lists eventually were reduced to a few more important activities with my daughter.

Which is a great lead-in to the next chapter.

Three
Still Be "You"

One of the enduring issues in the parenting of any child is the time or lack of time a parent gets to schedule for herself. Frustration develops when a parent, especially the main caregiver, rarely has time to engage in personally rewarding activities outside the home. Magnify this problem when caring for a child with disabilities since the time given in care usually increases. I found myself scheduling my outside activities during whatever time was "left over" or during the time I knew Katie was involved in school or work. My own part-time work schedule also complicated the issue. When Katie was quite small I learned a valuable lesson about caring for myself.

Through my church, I became acquainted with a friend who had a disability. "Joyce" cautioned me to never stop being me. She advised me to continue to pursue my own interests of education, tennis, and skiing. She punctuated this advice with her own sad story.

Apparently "Joyce's" mother gave up a promising career to become a full-time caregiver for her disabled daughter. Resentment grew. Once "Joyce" was able to care for herself, and, eventually to live independently, her mother ceased communication. Joyce had become the millstone around her mom's neck, the reason for her mother's lack of personal achievement. And her mother never forgave Joyce.

My conversation with "Joyce" was an epiphany for me,

and I realized the need to create and maintain my own sense of well-being. Admittedly, you need to juggle your needs with those of your child. This is not easy. Often it is discouraging. But it truly is important for your own mental and emotional sanity.

Whether you have certain life goals or dreams or whether you have an activity about which you are passionate or whether you just need time away, make time for yourself. The reason doesn't matter. What does matter is that this time gives you an outlet that somehow revitalizes you. To use hard-earned talents whether at work or in other activities may be your passion. Investigate the options that are available.

If you don't know how you would like to spend your time, then experiment. Start small. Take a class. There are many options in higher learning with flexible class schedules and online courses making it possible to pursue an education in bits and pieces. Exercise. Meet friends. Read a book. Shop. Volunteer. Just take care of yourself.

This "you" time does not miraculously appear. Planning must take place before it can ever happen. Once you have decided what you want to do, you must find an alternate caregiver and get the schedule on paper.

Finding helpful and trustworthy caregivers can be a hurdle. Because Katie is non-verbal, many capable young people were afraid to care for her, even for a few hours. This was very disheartening at times. Katie has had many caregivers through the years in the form of family, friends, neighbors, and agency personnel. The topic of choosing caregivers will be discussed in its own chapter. For now you need to understand that the effort you put into finding temporary caregivers will enhance your life and will probably enhance the lives of your child and of your family.

Next comes the scheduling. Gather all the information possible about your activity of interest, work with your caregiver's schedule, and coordinate the two. Most importantly once the plan is finalized put it on the calendar. Remember, you fought hard for this time. Don't let the opportunity go to waste through lack of communication.

Once Katie was on a regular school schedule and a schedule was coordinated with reliable caregivers, I was able to pursue many of my own interests. I found that I was and still am living life about a month in advance. Over time I have completed three additional college degrees. By learning to successfully schedule time, I was able to develop my own lifestyle and follow my dreams.

Yes, it can be frustrating. Things do not always fit in the schedule as planned. But persist in your efforts. You will find a source of respite. You owe it to yourself to not give up on you. You cannot be an effective and loving parent if you are not happy with who you are or with your situation.

Hi! My name is Katie. I am a special child with a disability, and there are some things that I cannot do. I cannot talk or write. But there are lots of things that I CAN do. I can swim, ride a bike, and go just about everywhere. What I do best is have fun.

My Mom has been the one to take care of me most of my life. Dad is around, but it is Mom who takes care of me. When I was younger I didn't like it very much when she would go away. Even staying with Dad just wasn't the same as being with Mom.

Often Mom would make arrangements for me to be involved in a program at a daycare center or a camp activity when she wanted or needed to do things for herself. Sometimes she would get a nice babysitter to stay with me. I have an aunt and uncle who have taken me to their house for a weekend but not very often.

As I got older and became more involved in school, the

more time Mom had to do her own things. Eventually I have gotten used to Mom not being with me all the time, partly because I can go and have fun at school or at daycare or at work. I am always happy to see Mom or Dad pick me up and to go home.

If I am home before Mom, I wait for her. Sometimes I sit by the window, sometimes I sit outside; sometimes I play outside and watch for her. Another thing that I do is to get ready all the things that I want to show her. I put my notebook from work and my projects on the counter so that they are ready as soon as Mom arrives.

Even though Mom isn't home to be with me all the time, I have learned how to still have fun!

Four

Help Your Children to Be Themselves

Defining your own interests can be complicated enough. An equally daunting task is to help your disabled child to develop his own interests and skills. Each child is an individual with personal likes, dislikes, and talents. What are they? And how do you find out?

Activities come in two categories: those you have tried and those you have not tried. Be open-minded about both. You may have to be involved in a wide variety of activities before your child finds one of interest. Don't force your own likes and preferences upon your child. Consider your child's abilities but don't set the bar too low. Let them stretch. Watch your child's reactions in both old and new situations. Pay attention to their facial expressions. The clues to how your child is responding to an activity will be visible. Watch for them.

You probably have a number of family activities that have become routine. Don't abandon any of them. Finding ways to include your child in these events may not be easy but be creative. Find the way that lets your child participate so that everyone is comfortable.

New activities provide new experiences. Some will work; some might not. The effort is always worth it. Take advantage of what your area has to offer. Call ahead to your local zoo or park or museum to see if they have any programs that might be of interest.

Katie taught our family much about her particular likes and dislikes. She did not always appreciate traditional holidays in the same way the rest of us did. Take Halloween for example. My son loved it! We all would get in costume, including the dog, and we just assumed that Katie would also enjoy the fun. We were all laughing, when we noticed that Katie was crying. What a shock it was when we realized that the dress-up frightened her to the point of making her physically ill. She was very interested in the candy, but petrified of the masks. It was even more traumatic that these ghosts and goblins who came to the door knew her name. She worked herself into an illness for days before Halloween even with the candy as an incentive.

Her fear of this holiday persisted until just a few years ago, when Katie was into her early twenties. She has finally allowed herself to dress in a totally benign outfit (a McDonald's shake) and will go to a select few of the neighbors' houses. Gradually, she has become confident enough to venture nearly the length of the entire street. But we have let her find her own level of involvement in Halloween. We had to back off, limit our own enthusiasm, and let her feel comfortable with this yearly event.

Katie's participation in another family activity had far more successful and enjoyable results but was totally unexpected. Her brother was a swimmer and had been on a swim team continuously since he was six years old. We would attend all his swim meets until he completed high school. One time, while we were at a pool, Katie just jumped in! Fully clothed! I guess she was trying to tell us something!

So we began the search for classes and instructors who would train her to be independent and safe in the water. In our town, the local YWCA offered one-on-one instruction. Katie "graduated" from this when she was able to propel herself the full length of the pool without assistance. It has taken many years, but she is now capable of swimming many lengths of the pool, and swims both freestyle and the backstroke. She practices weekly now and competes in the Special Olympics events—and she loves it.

Katie also loves to ski. I feel fairly sure that her interest was born of our interest. I think she wanted to be outdoors with us, rather than in a nursery for non-skiing children. It has taken years, but she is quite capable, and can ski almost anywhere with us.

We began to teach Katie to ski when she was about eight years old. We had saved Kent's outgrown ski equipment, and she had warm winter clothes. We took her to our "local" ski area, bought a lift ticket, and got out on the snow. She skied in between my legs for a bit, then on a tether, and then with a variety of braces that kept the tips of her skis from wandering.

Eventually we got Katie out to Breckenridge, Colorado, to the Breckenridge Outdoor Education Center (BOEC). They showed me some techniques to try ourselves. She also took lessons at the National Skiing Center for the Disabled (NSCD) at Winter Park, Colorado. She made great progress and gained much experience. Since then she has had many lessons at many ski areas in the United States and Canada.

Yes, it takes time. But you would do or already do the same for a "normal" child in your search to uncover their talents. There exists such a wide variety of opportunities, and it is your task to pursue this.

Although these were natural family events, Katie embraced them and took ownership of them.

*　　*　　*

Hi! My name is Katie. I am a very special child with a disability, and there are some things that I cannot do. I cannot

talk or write. But there are lots of things that I CAN do. What I do best is have fun.

I have an older brother named Kent who is a very good swimmer. He has been on many swim teams, and he always has liked to be in the water. I wanted to learn to like the water too.

There is a large swimming pool in my neighborhood. In the summer I like to go there to play in the water. But my parents did not want to worry about me all the time, so they tried to teach me how to swim.

At first I had "swimmies" on my arms. I was a little afraid to go in the deep water. Would they hold me up? They did! It was fun to kick and splash and still be safe.

Then I signed up for some swim lessons. Every week I went to the big pool, and a nice lady would stay with me. First I learned to kick my feet. Soon I learned how to stay afloat.

It has been hard for me to learn how to use my arms. I can't get them to move in big circles, but I can paddle. My instructors taught me how to swim the length of the pool.

But I am really good at swimming on my back. I look up at the sky, and I can kick very hard. I can go very fast this way.

I used to be unhappy about putting my face into the water. But I learned to hold my breath, and to even go under the water. Now I am not afraid to jump into deep water.

I am on a swim team for Special Olympics. I also was on the swim team for the country club. I have to go to many practices to be on the team. At practice we swim many lengths of the pool, sometimes using a kickboard. I get to practice, and it makes me stronger.

Being on the swim team means that I have to swim in races; sometimes I do a good job and swim the whole race. But sometimes I stop swimming and wave at everyone who is cheering. I know that is not what the coaches want, but the fans all look so happy.

I love to swim. I do not have as many trophies and ribbons as my brother Kent does, but I know I have just as much fun!

Besides swimming I like to snow ski. Everyone in my family likes to ski. My Mom and Dad have been skiing for a long time, and my brother Kent learned to ski when he as about six years old. I like to be with everyone and I like to be outside so I learned how to ski too.

It is very important to have the right equipment to ski. First, it is important to keep warm. I have my own snowsuit, or I wear a ski jacket and ski pants. I also have a warm hat, and warm ski mittens. And I wear long underwear, sweaters, and turtlenecks.

Every skier needs good-fitting ski boots. Warm socks need to fit inside the boot. These boots then fit onto skis, which for me, were very short when I learned and have gotten longer as I have gotten older.

When I was very little, my Mom would ski with me between her legs. She would help me get the feel of the snow. It was fun. As I grew, I was put into a harness. I would ski on my own but in front of my parents. This would keep me from going too fast.

Then I learned to ski next to my parents, with a brace on the tips of my skis. Soon I was able to ski all alone and to turn whenever I wanted. Now I only use a small bungee cord on the tips of my skis. The bungee cord is a stretchy but strong cord that is attached to the tips of each ski. It prevents my skis from crossing and gives me added stability when I am on a steep slope.

And I ski in Special Olympics, too! My Mom took me there because she was sure I could turn. It was a matter of turning around the gates on the course. The first year I just waved at everyone and didn't ski the course at all. I was disqualified. We went right home and didn't stay at the motel or anything. I was

18

upset. *I cried and did not want to go home. I was mad at my Mom.*

But the next winter I practiced more, and I did better. It is still a challenge to get me to pay attention to all the gates, but I am better. I have earned many medals now, and some of them are gold. I love going to the Ohio Special Olympics Winter Games.

I have been able to ski in lots of fun places. I usually ski in Michigan, but some of my best instructors have been in Colorado. I have flown in an airplane to take lessons at places like Breckenridge, Keystone, Copper Mountain, Winter Park, and the Big Mountain in Montana. There are many wonderful instructors everywhere.

I really like being outside, riding the chairlifts, and going down the slopes. I like to stop for lunch and watch others. It is a lot of fun!

Five

Be Affectionate

The personal inventory is not over yet. Not only do you need to consider your own attitudes about disability and account for your own desires and needs, but you must also take stock of your emotional makeup. Become aware of how you express affection.

Giving physical love to the child with disabilities can sometimes be a challenge. First, emotional barriers may exist. Some of these barriers may be tied up in your own attitudes. After all, this is not the "perfect" child that you thought you were going to raise. This punctuates the need to really examine any preconceptions that you may have. Your own upbringing may be a barrier to the expression of affection. Consider whether you openly express your feelings in a physical way or whether your expression is more reserved.

Secondly, a child's own physical difficulties may create barriers. Life support apparatus and mobility equipment all make it difficult to just give the child a hug. Never lose sight that the child exists in the middle of all the mechanical structures. Again, creative thinking helps to overcome these obstacles.

Any barriers to the physical expression of love can be broken down. Touch is a means of communicating with your child. It both expresses sentiment and provides instruction. The importance of touch takes on greater significance with a child who has difficulty with verbal communication. I have read that to merely exist an individual needs twelve hugs a day.

Touch can strengthen your bond with your child. For the child it establishes a link to the world. The benefits of this are that she will be more willing to explore with you, will try to achieve and learn new things, and will feel proud of her own accomplishments. This will build her self-esteem and give her the confidence to face the already uncertain world. She could already be aware that she is somehow different. Touch imparts acceptance, gives value, and builds self-esteem.

Remember that as the caregiver you are the teacher for the rest of the family and the rest of the community. Others will follow your example. Touch gives credence to being a valued member of your family and a valued member of society.

Fortunately for me, the physical constraints were never a part of life with Katie. After she learned to walk, being with her, in close contact with her, was always the scenario. This was not problematic as I was taught to be a parent who is not afraid to express love to my children. I was always affectionate even in public with both my children. We often were involved in tickling, snuggling, and hugging.

My son began a ritual game which we call "I'm next to Mommy." Usually at night before bedtime when we were all bathed and in our night clothes, Katie would sit next to me in my bed as I read, and sometimes she would fall asleep or at least get ready to sleep there. Son Kent, when in junior high, would "invade" the space, and try to get in between Katie and me. If he succeeded in squeezing himself between us, Katie would get upset and run around to the other side of the bed to my other side. Of course, Kent would try to change sides too. Amidst tons of laughter, the bed was disheveled, and no one was ready for bed anymore.

We also were fond of group hugs, where Katie was the

21

"in-between" part of the hug. Affection is very important to self-acceptance. Don't be afraid to show it and the benefits will become apparent in the confidence to explore that will be developed in your child.

*   *   *

Hi! My name is Katie. I am a special child with a disability, and there are some things that I cannot do. I cannot talk or write. But there are lots of things that I CAN do. I can swim, ride a bike, go skiing and go just about everywhere. What I do best is have fun.

I am a pretty lucky girl, because I know that I am loved. Of course, I encourage this because I like to give and get hugs. It started at home with lots of hugs being given at our house.

My brother Kent is older than I am. When my Mom would go to his school to help out with lunch or something, she was always sneaking up on him to give him a hug. I guess he liked it because he was always giving her hugs back.

He also started the "I'm next to Mommy" game. At night, when I have had my bath, and am all snuggled up with a book with Mom at my side, Kent would come into the bedroom and try to take away my spot next to her! Since he was bigger and stronger, he would usually wiggle his way into the bed between us. It made me SO angry!! I would get frustrated and try to run around the other side of the bed to get to Mom's other side, but then he would go there too!! I was never fast enough!

Now that I am older, I still like to be next to Mommy, and sometimes Kent still teases me with that. But in the end, I know both Mommy and Kent love me. They give me lots of hugs, and we have fun.

Six

Be a Parent: Be Firm, Be Consistent

Did I just say, "Learn how to be tender with your child"? In expressing your love for your child, touch and tenderness must be used. Yet when it comes to teaching your child, I will encourage you to stand like a rock and be a firm disciplinarian.

When Katie was under five years old, I received a valuable piece of advice. A friend, an older parent with grown children, advised me to be firm. Just because Katie was disabled was no reason to make excuses for her behavior or allow her to get away with behaviors that were unacceptable. In other words, I was advised to be a parent.

Studies in psychology reveal that authoritative parenting is most successful. This style of parenting calls for firm consistent expectations to be set for the child with the result being a competent individual who is aware of parental love and concern. Communication of these guidelines is most important along with the follow through. It calls for consequences for both good and bad behavior. As the child grows and becomes more independent, she gradually assumes more responsibility for her actions. These same concepts apply to parenting the disabled. Behavioral expectations should be established, and consequences should follow.

You, the parent, are the only unchanging variable in the life of your child. It is up to you to set the example by being firm and consistent. It is not easy. Your child will not always like your decisions. But that is your job.

I soon realized my friend was right. The phrase "doesn't know any better" only applies if you have never made the effort to teach acceptable behavior. Even though Katie was non-verbal, my husband and I knew that she understood our conversation and was well aware of her actions. Often she would try to use her disability to get "away with murder."

In our case, we decided that parenting Katie was going to be no different than parenting Kent. The same rules for behavior were applied and expected. Katie has always been held to the same behavioral standards.

Too often, parents of the disabled refuse to outline the rules and to establish guidelines for behavior. Some parents are too weak and afraid to be parents, and do not challenge their child to a high standard of behavior. Some parents of those with a disability feel sorry for their child and never set guidelines for behavior. The rules of parenting are the same as for normal children. Working with your child with disabilities will take more time, and the results will not be immediate. The timetable will be different, and it can get discouraging. But all family members should attempt to be on the same page with the same set of expectations. The results will be worth it.

This is not easy. Parenting is not easy. It will take longer and will take more effort. It is ongoing. Know that with children with a disability, the goal of independence may never be reached, but do not abdicate your responsibility as a loving parent who has the best interest of your child at heart.

I beg you, do not say that "She is disabled so it is okay if she sits in front of the TV and eats potato chips all day," or "She can act out in anger." Set expectations. Follow through. Be firm.

*   *   *

Hi! My name is Katie. I am a very special child with a disability, and there are some things that I cannot do. I cannot talk or write. But there are lots of things that I CAN do. What I do best is have fun.

One of that places that I have had fun in my life is at school, riding the bus every day, and now, going to work. I have been very lucky that my parents, especially my mom, have tried hard to do the best for me. When I was only five years old, Mom had to go to a school board meeting to get permission for me to go to school. I had to be tested with a book that had a lot of pictures in it. I must have passed, because I got to go to school!

The first day of school I got to ride the bus. Mom took pictures of me that first time I got on the bus and the first time I came home. Through the years when I have been in a special school program, like a play or physical education presentation, Mom came to take pictures of me.

Over the years, I have had some fun bus drivers too. Most of my drivers have had a great sense of humor, have remembered my birthday, and have given me little presents on holidays. Now I ride the bus to work every day, and it still is fun.

Seven
Behavior Modification

If guiding behavior was just a matter of being firm and consistent in your approach to your child, then the whole process would be easy. Sorry. Behavior is a function of myriad internal and external influences. Include your child's personality and type and level of disability in those influences, and you can begin to see how specialized this task can be for each child. Add to the mix a spectrum of possible language complications. Being able to understand conversation, receptive language, might be in place but a lack of ability to express oneself (expressive language) adds to the complexity of the situation.

Even defining what is good behavior and what is bad behavior can be unclear. For example, elbows on the table during a meal may cause one family to wilt with shame while another family may consider it to be an everyday activity expressing relaxation and comfort. My point here is that as with everything else in your child's life you must be the one to set the standard and define what is acceptable and what is not. You are the most important participant in your child's behavioral formation.

Forgive me if I begin to sound clinical here but shaping behavior is a multiple step process. Let me try to organize this information.

1. Understand your child's current behavior. Observe

them. Try to determine why they act as they do. If your child lacks verbal skills, then observation is key.

2. Know your child's physical and emotional capabilities. Stretching a child's potential is the goal; asking the impossible is devastating.

3. Know what your expectations are. Don't be vague about the behavior you want to see. No one can work towards a goal if they do not understand what it is.

4. Communicate with all involved. The wanted behavior should be encouraged in all the child's settings. Talk with all other family members, teachers, and caregivers about what you are working towards and what their roles should be.

5. Plan. Know how you want to go about achieving the desired behavior. This involves communicating with all key people. Also know what the consequences should be if the behavior is not followed. Be consistent and persistent.

6. Re-evaluate. Is your approach working? Have you given your plan enough time? Did you raise the bar to high or not high enough? Build your evaluation questions into your plan of action so that you know ahead of time what criteria you will use to evaluate the progress.

During Katie's early years, we were given little or no professional advice on how to manage behavior. I was guided by my experience in education, in the classroom. But since we were determined to have her with us and involved in the family activities her behavior became a factor. Once we determined her level of understanding, we worked on communicating the behavior we expected. Taking into consideration her developmental delays, the methods we used to train Katie were no different than what we used on our son. Watching her closely gave us indications as to how well she understood or could react to a situation.

When school started for Katie, her behavior was monitored through a system of handwritten communications with her teachers. Katie would come home each day with a folder containing detailed forms that the teacher would have completed. Every day we were updated on what had transpired at school. We mirrored this process at home by recording her daily activities there, and returning this to school. These forms documented what she ate, how she behaved, what her activities were, etc. This process helped us to understand Katie at school, and it helped the teacher to understand Katie at home.

Eventually the form letter gave way to a notebook, a spiral pad of sorts that traveled back and forth. There was no set formula for conversation, no exact specifics from day to day, but we were able to keep tabs on her behavior. The only regularly scheduled meetings between the teacher and parents came when the yearly Individualized Education Plan (IEP) meeting took place. The IEP is a government document that is a collaborative effort to set goals for and monitor the progress of your child.

Because Katie has always been a cheerful and healthy individual, her behavior for most of her life has been pleasant and flexible. Katie exudes a positive attitude and an excitement for life that is infectious. She has an innate desire to learn new behavior and to adopt behavior that pleases others. Whenever she learns a new skill we slap "high fives" and give "thumbs up." The development of a new behavior is exciting, but remember that the development of the behavior could take time. Be cautious in your expectations.

Rehearsing good behavior before an event is a useful technique that might benefit a child. Preparing ahead of time and building the expected behavior before the situation happens could prevent unwanted behavior.

Know that modifying behavior is an ongoing process. The onset of puberty and the hormonal changes that accompany it can bring changes in temperament and therefore behavior. Katie was much more easygoing and predictable before puberty. Consult with your physician for possible suggestions and the best advice at this time.

Management of Katie's behavior makes it easier to keep her with us, but as we realized early on behavior also was a safety issue. Safety can be a concern with both good and bad behavior. For example, Katie is a very friendly person. Her instinct is to greet everyone she meets with hugs as if she knows them all. Trying to hug strangers can create problems so to this day we constantly work to teach Katie the behavior of shaking hands. It is a goal at work and in her speech classes at The University of Toledo.

Behavior has always been an issue with Katie. She does have negative behaviors that have been a continuous challenge. Her negative behavior stems, we think, from her frustration with an issue or situation. She will begin by striking herself on the head, and it could escalate into hitting others, biting herself or others, or throwing herself on the ground and refusing to walk. Because she is non-verbal, and can only make sounds, we have no way of knowing what is bothering her, or what her reason is for inappropriate acts. We have tried to deal with it in a variety of ways over the years. These are outlined below.

Her teachers tried very hard to keep track of days when her behavior was unacceptable. We communicated about the possible reasons for this and developed a system of rewards for good days. It helped communication between the adults, at least.

At her work place, we have a very structured behavior plan of action for the times when she misbehaves. As always safety is an issue since there is a concern that Katie could hurt herself or hurt others. A chart has been made for each day of the week and divided into three times of day. Her goal is to receive three stickers each day. This comes home at the end of the week and is posted on the refrigerator. I am not sure if it is entirely effective, but at least it lets Katie know that when her behavior is unacceptable, we will all know it and have a conversation about it. The behavior is discussed at home, with appropriate rewards or punishments, and the behavior is a topic of discussion in our twice yearly meetings to plan Katie's continued care and work plans.

*   *   *

Hi! My name is Katie. I am a very special child with a disability, and there are lots of things that I cannot do. I cannot talk or write. But there are lots of things that I CAN do. What I do best is have fun.

Since I cannot say words, I sometimes have a difficult time expressing how I feel. When I am happy, I often cheer by making a "yeah"ing sound, and I wave my arms in the air. I see people acting this way at sporting events, and I do the same thing. Everyone around me knows when I am excited!

When I am angry or upset, I also let everyone know. I can get very sad and cry when I see things around me that I don't like or when I am hurt. Usually mom tries to comfort me, and I can settle down.

But when I am angry, I hit myself and sometimes others too. My teachers and now the people I work with don't want me to hurt myself or others. They try to get me alone and get me to calm down by taking deep breaths. I am sorry afterwards, and I can say in sign language that I am sorry.

Sometimes at home I have to go to my room. I don't like it, and I find it hard to stay there and I cry. This is a time when I definitely do not have fun.

Eight
Modifying Parents' Behavior

Parents must realize that occasionally it is their behavior that requires modification because often their own behavior may trigger a reaction in their child.

Because Katie's listening or "receptive" language is so good, we have developed our own system of communication between ourselves as parents and have modified our behavior around Katie.

In order to deal with Katie's particular temperament and level of understanding, we have developed a few guidelines for communication.

1. We DO NOT disclose information about a future trip or event too far in advance! Katie has little sense of time. If the information gets out that we are going on a trip, she expects immediate action. There have been some negative behaviors emanating from her when the event did not happen in the fashion "advertised" or in a timely manner. Since we don't understand her thinking, making the situation clear to her is next to impossible. We have experienced "meltdowns" while at Sea World and Disneyworld when the line for a ride was too long or a show closed and we needed to readjust our plans.

2. We DO NOT say something we don't think she

should hear. We have found that remarks made in casual conversation initiate action on her part. She often overhears a guest indicate a need for an ash tray or that they should be getting home now. The ash tray magically appears or the correct coat comes out of the closet and is given to the guest. Just because she does not talk does not mean that she isn't listening.

3. We DO NOT talk about her as if she cannot hear. These remarks can be devastating and diminish her self-esteem. She finds arguments particularly disturbing.

Other types of disabilities may require different strategies. Again being aware of your own child's capabilities will help you to make changes in your own behavior when needed. Some children with a disability may need a time of rehearsal, or much advanced conversation. This does not help in our situation.

*   *   *

Hi! My name is Katie. I am a very special child with a disability, and there are some things that I cannot do. I cannot talk or write. But there are lots of things that I CAN do. What I do best is to have fun.

I really like to go places with my family and with my caregivers. They will tell me about a place or an activity, and sometimes I get very excited! I may not understand when that activity is going to take place. I think I get too anxious to go. It is good that I like to do things, but I can be a handful.

One time when we were at Disneyworld, we had to change our plans because a bus was too full. I got very upset! My behavior was very inappropriate! I even sat down on the ground and refused to move. I have a hard time with sudden change.

Eventually another bus came, and we all got to go to the Park. But I was bad, and I don't always understand how things work. I think I get my mind set on what we are to do, and I don't listen to how it is really going to happen.

But I am pretty good most of the time. Besides, that is how I can have fun.

Nine

Language

Nothing can be accomplished with behavior or anything else if you cannot communicate with your child. Your communication can be verbal or visual or tactile; it does not matter. What does matter is that the communication conveys a message, a message that is understood. The number of physical and mental barriers present will determine how complicated this communication process can be.

Communication with Katie is a big issue. She is unable to say words though she can and does make some sounds. She can say "momma" and a few other "almost" words. In spite of numerous tests and interventions, Katie's speech never progressed much beyond the level of an infant. Slowly it became apparent that she was never going to speak full words.

When Katie started primary school, she was most fortunate to have a teacher, Kelly, who taught the class sign language. Kelly taught children with a variety of disabilities and tried to use sign language to reach as many as she could. She was very firm. For the first time in her life, Katie was able to initiate conversation through signing (expressive language) as well as respond to questions using signing (receptive language).

After a few years in school, Kelly encouraged us to investigate the use of a speech board, a talking device. This device has icons that when pressed would say the word or sentence.

In this way, Katie was able to initiate conversation, ask questions, and respond in many ways. She began with a very rudimentary board and over the years has upgraded to a more sophisticated device that offers many speech opportunities. Her first board was very large, about the size of a "See and Say" toy. She learned to use it very rapidly and we had it reprogrammed several times. As the technology improved, the size of the device decreased, while the number of functions has increased. To this day Katie still uses her board. It is utilized mainly at work, but it is also programmed for many social activities.

There are a wide variety of augmentation communication products available. Additionally technological advances have made these devices smaller, less expensive, and easier to use. The most comprehensive catalog for devices that I have seen comes from Saltillo Corporation. They can be reached at 1–800–382–8622 by telephone or online at www.saltillo.com.

Even with new technologies on our side, we often do not understand what is going on with Katie, and her frustrations come out. We struggle to understand what situations cause her to get upset. At these times, we quickly intervene, try to calm her down, and re-direct her attention to another situation.

One of the neat things about Katie is that she usually adapts. She has always been attentive to her surroundings, and been observant when we have company or she is out. Sometimes she recognizes a need or a situation before we do. Although she learned the standard sign language in her elementary years, she has then made up signs of her own. She has invented her own signs for certain events, people and activities.

For example, we had an Uncle who always liked to tickle her and roughhouse when he came over. I am sure it would have been too tedious to spell out the words "Uncle Bob," so when she wanted to inquire about him, she would tickle her armpit. We have another friend who is allowed to smoke in our house. Katie's sign for him is to put her fingers up to her mouth and blow on them.

In similar fashion, she has developed her own signs for tennis, swimming, skiing, baseball, and a number of other activities. I guess that is her intelligence showing, and we all know what she is talking about. This innovation on her part has allowed her to initiate a "conversation" about a sport or an event. It is like she is asking a question, and surely makes it easier for her to make her needs known.

Continue to explore communication options that meet or can enhance your child's needs. New equipment and ideas are always hitting the market.

*   *   *

Hi! My name is Katie. I am a very special child with a disability, and there are some things that I cannot do. I cannot talk or write. But there are lots of things that I CAN do. But what I do best is to have fun.

It is a bit frustrating to have something to say and not to be able to say it. I have lots of questions about who the company might be, or what the activity might be, or what we are going to eat. So sometimes I make up a sign that looks like the activity or reminds me of the person.

Most of the time it works out great but one time I think my parents were kind of embarrassed. I really like pizza! So I make up a triangle shape with my fingers and thumbs. I was so proud of it! One time I used it at Church with a lady who taught sign language. She laughed at me! I was told that the sign I used is really supposed to mean "vagina"—whatever that is.

But my parents taught me the right sign for pizza, and now that is what I use. That is fun.

Ten

Caregivers

You will need help in giving care to your child. Try to accept this, get comfortable with it, and plan for it. Be aware that this is not a personal failing or weakness but a necessity. Realizing that doing all that is required of you is not easy and utilizing outside resources that are available to you will provide benefits for you, your family, and your child.

The first reason to seek the assistance of caregivers is you. If a parent never spends time away from her child, then the rest of the world has a hard time assigning value to the parent outside of the caregiver role. We have talked already about the need to structure personal time for yourself either to achieve your life goals or merely for respite and relaxation. Considering this to be a priority in your life is crucial. This point cannot be stressed enough.

The second reason to utilize a caregiver is to give your other family some individual attention. Besides the primary caregiver needing personal time, other members of the family will also need some respite from time to time. Plan a date with your spouse or a play date with your other children or have a special afternoon or meal together. Because a special child comes into your life does not mean that the rest of your world disappears. Others will still need your specialized individual attention.

The third reason to surround yourself with other caregivers concerns the benefits that your child will reap. Too often, and my case is no exception, a parent falls into the trap of knowing that no one can provide the same level of quality care that she can. Consequently, the child never learns to rely on anyone else, never learns to trust anyone else. The end product of such a closed system is a child who is far too dependent on the parent, and a parent who cannot ever break away. Part of the reason that you will want to do this is to let your child get used to the care of other good people.

Caregivers are utilized in two separate settings. In one situation the caregiver comes to your home. The home caregiver may come occasionally to babysit so that you can get a day out or may come on a more permanent basis so that you can get to work every day. The other setting is located outside the home constituting a variety of places. Schools, daycare agencies, clubs, state agencies, and churches are some of the outside organizations that may offer care for your child. Out of the home situations will be discussed under the heading of *Respite/Camps*.

Because Katie was so perpetually happy and at ease with people, finding a caregiver while she was an infant was somewhat simple. When I left the home both of my children needed a sitter and a variety of local teenagers were available and willing. I was fortunate that I knew the kids available in the area before they came. Input from my son helped determine the value of the sitter and helped me decide whether they should be asked to return. If the sitter was good enough for Kent, she was good enough for Katie.

When Katie had her brother around she was always accepting of other people, caregivers included; but the situation changed when she was home alone. Whenever I would begin to leave, Katie would become distressed. This developed because she had become so dependent on me.

Perhaps the most difficult situation we faced was the daily

routine of getting on and off the bus. Normally my work schedule allowed me to be present for the bus send off and drop off. When I got a full-time office job, I no longer could be available. We had to arrange for a caregiver to be at the house in time for the afternoon bus. If Katie sensed I was not there, she would refuse to get off the bus. Katie completely rejected the caregiver making for a difficult situation. When I did get home, Katie would say "good-bye" and show the caregiver to the door.

For a caregiver to gain the trust of a child with disabilities can be a tough assignment. We have "gone through" three different caregivers. We have done much better in the last years. Katie is fortunate to have a wonderful caregiver who takes no nonsense, yet handles Katie with affection. With her help, Katie often prepares simple meals (spaghetti sauce), makes cookies or brownies, folds laundry, and sets the table. Getting to this point was not easy. The firm yet patient approach of the caregiver has helped Katie learn new skills. Some tasks still only happen with the caregiver's assistance. But Katie has developed a sense of pride in accomplishing the tasks for the day. Be prepared for some disappointments, but perseverance definitely pays off for both the parent and the child.

*   *   *

Hi! My name is Katie. I am a very special child with a disability, and there are things that I cannot do. I cannot talk or write. But there are lots of things that I CAN do. What I do best is have fun.

A real problem for me was learning how to work with people other than my Mom. I did not have fun when I was learning to be with another caregiver. I even acted badly and was unkind.

I have become comfortable with babysitters since I was

little. But the days when Mom wasn't there to meet my bus, I really was upset. When I could see the other lady, I would cry, and throw my book bag, and sit down on the bus steps. I refused to get off of the bus.

After a while, things did get better, and I realized that this person wanted to have fun with me too. And she was pretty good at it. Over the last couple of years I have learned to get used to several good caregivers. They have taught me how to fold clothes, how to make my bed, how to set the table, how to do some of the cooking and baking, and how to make some of the foods that I love.

My current caregiver Marita also takes me to fun places. We go to the park; we play Putt-Putt, we go swimming and shopping and do lots of other things. So I have learned that caregivers are also people who want to have fun. And we do.

Eleven
Respite/Camps

Taking the child with a disability out of the safe and familiar home environment and leaving them in the care of other people in a not-so-familiar setting can have its own set of problems and benefits.

Unfamiliarity with the surroundings and the personnel can cause a child to become upset. Perhaps the child is used to being the center of attention and the focus of all activity. In the new setting, the child needs to learn to share time and space with others.

So by taking the child out of a vacuum, she learns better how to adapt to new environments and accept new people. Everyone grows by exposure to new life experiences and the child with a disability is no different.

How much respite care often depends on the demands of the parents' jobs, the season of the year, and the number of remaining responsibilities, such as other children, or elderly family members who need care. The severity of the child's disability also is a factor.

The type and variety of respite care varies in every location. Information concerning these opportunities does not come easily. Sifting through the yellow pages, talking to a case worker, going online, or information handed out at school are a few of the ways you can get information about available care. The more effort you invest, the better the results.

On the rare occasion that two programs were operating at the same time, the choice was made based on family schedules and financial considerations. Our goal was to expose Katie to as many different educational experiences as possible.

We found county programs that operate under the umbrella of the Association for Retarded Citizens, and these operate year round. This one organization led us to more opportunities throughout the years. Local and county offices for Mental Retardation/Developmental Delays (MR/DD) as well as sheltered workshops for those capable of work can be found in the telephone book. There are Special Olympics organizations in every state and camps and programs designed for specific disabilities. Our experiences with the YMCA have been fantastic over the years. Katie was able to participate in YMCA programs until she turned eighteen years old. In fact, many of the camp experiences and day care opportunities are offered for specific age groups only.

Educators and child care experts alike agree that keeping children busy and on a schedule is a good thing. Summer became the most challenging time in which to keep Katie busy because school was out of session and our work schedules continued. In Katie's case, she does well with a schedule and likes life to be predictable. The task was to identify activities that Katie would like, and learn from, as she went through her summer days.

Finding information about available summer or camp opportunities came from individual research and flyers from school. Over the years, there has been a more concerted effort to educate parents about the variety of services available in our area. There have been "parent fairs" where the various agencies, camps, and programs are on display and have information available. It is a great help.

In our local area, there is a wonderful organization that offers a variety of services for all levels of disability, Sunshine

Inc. This facility is situated on about six acres of land and provides full-time living arrangements for people whose disabilities vary in type and severity. Weekend activities are also offered for those who still live at their own home and want to participate in activities with their peers. Sometimes the activities involve a short trip (to a ball game, a park, or a boat ride), and sometimes they engage in crafts on the grounds.

When Katie was between six and twelve years of age, this facility and others offered day camp experiences. Most of the camps operated for a "session" and these times varied from all day and for many weeks, to portions of days for just one week. Additionally, as Katie grew in age and ability, the local YMCA also found a place for Katie during their summer sessions. The Y programs offered her and others like her an opportunity to interact with "normal" children in a wide variety of activities and outings.

We have also found a few overnight camps that Katie loves. She now feels comfortable at a camp close to home where she has spent several weekends. We also have located a camp in the next state where Katie has been going for fifteen years. She is often so excited upon arrival that she flings open the car door before we can park.

The only downside for the working parent is that at some point many of these wonderful programs have age limit requirements making a child ineligible. Most of the camps advertise the age limit for their clientele. For us, it was indeed a sad day when the YMCA finally was required to cut Katie from their programs.

*   *   *

Hi! My name is Katie. I am a very special child with a disability, and there are some things that I cannot do. I cannot

talk or write. But there are lots of things that I CAN do. What I do best is have fun.

When I was a little girl, my parents wanted me to be in school. They had to find a special class for me. It was a nice class where there were many special kids. Some were not able to walk and were in wheelchairs; some needed a walker. Some could not see very well; some were like me and could not talk.

My Mom was a little worried about me going to school, because I had to ride a yellow bus. I loved it! I watched my brother and all the other kids in the neighborhood get on a bus, and I was really excited to do it too.

I have very special drivers and bus aides. They are all very nice to me. They know I am excited to be with them.

I am so excited to go to school that I get up early every morning just to be sure that I am ready on time. While I eat my breakfast, I watch out the window to see the bus. When I spot it coming around the corner, I get my coat on, pick up my back-pack, and head out the door. Mom or Dad always walks me to the bus.

Going to school helps me to learn lots of things. We are working with numbers, letters, and money. Sometimes I get to do jobs for the teacher like take notes to the office. I never get lost. Sometimes we fold papers or go to places to try a job. If we are at school, we clean the tables in the cafeteria as our job. Sometimes we go on a field trip, to the zoo or to a movie or to the park.

The counselors at camp help me take care of myself. They help me with the shower and with washing my hair. They help me keep track of my clothes and to take lots of pictures of what I do at camp. They are great to put in my picture album.

On Friday morning, Mom returns to take me home. I am usually tired when I come home. I often fall asleep in the car. But I usually wait until after we stop for an ice cream treat—one more way to have fun.

Twelve

Vacations

It has been said that a "trip" is when the family travels together, and a "vacation" is the time when the parents can travel alone. Although I think that for some families this is true, I tend to think that any amount of time I am able to get away from the routine and just be in a different environment is a vacation to me. It is definitely important to plan for time away from home both with and without your child with disabilities.

As an infant Katie went with us everywhere. By the time we learned she had a disability she had already been traveling with us for eighteen to twenty months. Hence she expected to travel with us anywhere that we went. For the most part, this is not a major problem, because Katie is so high functioning and is able to do many things for herself. She understands the circumstances of events. When our family was invited to visit friends at a cottage, Katie came along. When we went on a picnic or to a county fair, Katie came along. When we would go boating, she came along. She truly traveled virtually everywhere with us.

Often it is a challenge to locate a vacation spot that can accommodate a disabled child. The type and severity of the disability can also make arranging for a vacation more complex. As with all other activities, planning ahead of time is the key to a successful vacation.

For Katie, I believe taking her with us to so many places has assisted her in developing a sense of belonging and self thereby adding to her identity within the family. We live with a camera "at the ready" and have very large family albums. When Katie looks through the albums and sees herself in all the activities and adventures, she smiles and becomes excited. She often shows an album to a guest, finds herself in a picture, and points to the picture and then to herself. These are wonderful moments.

Katie loves to fly! Although it has been several years since her first flight (probably to a ski resort), she continues to be excited about the prospect of air travel. She is excited to go, always gets the seat by the window, and cheers when we lift off and land. Her enthusiasm is really quite refreshing.

Since we have mostly treated Katie as just a normal member of the traveling party, we never made a big deal of air travel. We neither expected nor received any special treatment. If a child has more severe disabilities and needs physical accommodations then the airline should be contacted ahead of time so that arrangements can be made.

There have been a few occasions when my husband and I have traveled without children. Travel abroad is one of those times. If we knew that we would be involved in a great deal of walking or would encounter language changes in foreign countries, then we opted to leave both children at home. Although these situations are not the norm, it can be nice to have a true "vacation."

Probably the key to travel is to be aware of the limitations of your child. Plan for them or plan around them. Do not underestimate the benefits you, your child, and your family will get from travel.

*　　*　　*

Hi! My name is Katie. I am a very special child with a disability, and there are some things that I cannot do. I cannot talk or write. But there are lots of things that I CAN do. What I do best is to have fun.

This is about my trip to an island. An island is a place that is surrounded by water. The only way to get there is on a boat.

Many things have to be taken care of before we can go. First, I had to help pack my clothes for the trip, since I could not just go to my room for more clothes. I had to pack clothes for warm weather and clothes for cool weather.

Then we had to plan what food to take. We packed a big cooler with all the things we needed to cook. We put lots of ice in the cooler just before we closed it.

I have two dogs, and we had to pack for them too! I made sure that we had their leashes, dog bones, and food. They like trips too.

We put everything in the car and drove to the ferry. It is a big boat that has room for cars, trucks, and people. At the dock, strong ropes hold the boat to the dock so that everyone and everything can get on. A man tells us when to drive the car on, and Dad is careful to follow his directions. Even with the tight ropes, the boat is moving a little. It is exciting.

When the boat is ready to leave, a very loud horn sounds. It scares me, and I cover my ears. Once the boat leaves the dock, we can get out of the car and walk around on deck. The dogs have to stay on leashes.

Usually it is a nice ride to the island. Sometimes it is rough and the waves splash up on the boat. I stay away from the waves.

Often there are other small boats on the lake. I wave at the people on all of them. Sometimes they wave back.

When we get to the island, the horn blows loudly again. Then the strong ropes are tied and we can drive off of the ferry. It is a great way to have fun.

Thirteen
Public Exposure

How much public exposure you and your child with disabilities want must be considered. Think about two questions. How do you as the parent feel about your child in public? And how do you think your child feels about functioning in the public eye?

The possibility could exist that either parent or child is in some way ashamed of or diminished by the disability. Honestly examine this issue perhaps with professional help or with the assistance of a parenting group.

Consider too the amount of stimulation the child can absorb successfully. Just as infants can become overstimulated with too much attention or too much activity around them, the child with disabilities might be overcome by a situation in which there is just too much going on. If appropriate behavior is an issue for the child, too much attention in the public arena can be a cause for acting out. If this is the case then it may take time to develop a level of comfort in public situations. Some level of comfort can be achieved by working on this problem slowly.

I think the days are gone when a child with a disability is hidden away and is not exposed to the "real world." Certainly our educational system in the United States has passed laws in an effort to accommodate students with disabilities. These laws have made it possible for students with disabilities to function in a regular school and pursue as "normal" a life as is possible. In my limited experience, classes are held within a regular school, and they give the students with disabilities many opportunities to interact with the rest of the student body.

Inclusion in school activities is something that probably varies from one school system to another and from one grade level to another. It has been our experience that many of Katie's teachers have tried to involve her class in many school-wide activities. In her elementary years, the holiday parties, parades, and festivities were always inclusive. The special needs classes were included in school presentations.

Katie's teachers were in close contact with us regarding each of the public events. We discussed how much participation we felt would be good for Katie. She is very much a "people person" so there have been very few constraints put on her activities. The only exception over the years has been to limit the level of participation in events centered on Halloween since Katie has a problem with some of the costumes.

To show support for Katie and for the teachers who worked so hard to provide varied experiences for our daughter, we tried to attend every event that we could.

Because Katie could ski, she was considered a member of the ski club at her high school. There were a few trips scheduled every year, and Katie often participated in the one-day trips to the ski areas nearby. It was a real ego boost for her to be recognized on the slopes by individuals who were only used to seeing her in the school environment. In fact, because of her skiing ability, she could often perform better on skis than many of the "regular" students. And they did not hesitate to point this out making Katie feel very good about herself and her skills.

Perhaps the most difficult decision along these lines was whether or not Katie should participate in high school graduation. At first I thought it would not be a good idea especially since the ceremony would take place in a very public theater. I was worried about Katie's behavior and I did not want to place her in a situation where she might be ridiculed.

We were encouraged by her teachers to have her be a part of the ceremony. Ultimately she and we decided that she would participate. It was great fun! She wore her cap and gown, knew exactly how to walk across the stage, and handled herself in a manner befitting a high school graduate. For her and for us it was a wonderful event to complete her years of formal schooling.

As with all other situations, whether a child participates in events or not is based on an individual assessment of the child's abilities.

*   *   *

Hi! My name is Katie. I am a very special child with a disability, and there are some things that I cannot do. I cannot talk or write. But there are lots of things that I CAN do. What I do best is to have fun.

When I was finishing my "senior year" at high school, all the other seniors were getting their pictures taken and doing special things for graduation. My mom wasn't so sure just how much we were going to do, but in the end, we did lots!

The fall before graduation I posed for my senior pictures just like all the other students. Mom made an appointment, and I got to pick out my clothes. I wore my favorite sweater, and we took along some of the reminders of things I like to do. Then we had time to put me in different poses, and they took lots of pictures. Only one of them went in the yearbook, but then we had the others to give to people.

The picture that was in the yearbook was just of my face and shoulders. But the other pictures were taken with me and my swim goggles and another few with my Special Olympics medals. We chose one pose for a nice picture to put on our bookcase and then another pose for some wallet sizes to hand out. Now my high school picture is on the bookcase just like my brother. And everyone can see how much fun I have.

Fourteen
Acknowledge Successes

Everyone likes to be recognized for an accomplishment. A child with disabilities is no exception. The achievements may not come as often. They may not seem monumental to the public eye. But to the child with disabilities each step forward is gained only with effort and perseverance and is deserving of public acknowledgement. Parents recognize their child's successes, no matter how big or small. Use these moments to foster pride and encourage potential future growth.

As Katie has grown up, there have been a variety of opportunities for praise. Early in her schooling, awards were given for achieving an otherwise easily aquired skill. "Best Student" awards often were brought home. Katie was once recognized as the "Most Enthusiastic Swimmer" on her swim team, as the "Best Break Dancer" at a Christmas Party, or more recently, as the "Employee of the Month" at work. Everyone on her baseball or bowling teams receives a trophy, and she is proud of these.

When these awards come home, we always make a big deal over them. Ribbons and certificates are placed on the refrigerator; her trophies and medals adorn the bookshelves. She has been featured in the newspapers over the years. The articles are laminated and placed on the refrigerator or in Katie's room.

Special Olympics is an excellent organization that pays

homage to the participation of each individual—win or lose. Each entrant receives an award of some sort. Although all competitors receive awards, honor is also given to those who place first, second, or third in their respective sports. These awards are definitely arranged in descending order recognizing the winners with medals. For some of the people with disabilities, just being able to participate is enough. Only those who develop a more keen sense of competition recognize the difference in the award and truly strive to be the best in their event.

At this point in Katie's life, she definitely recognizes the difference between a medal and a ribbon. When the Olympics are televised and the athletes are awarded their medals, Katie feels a deep kinship with them. She often retrieves her medals from the book case and puts them on again. She too has achieved. She shares in their accomplishments, and she perceives that they share in hers.

Sports have provided Katie with opportunities to strive and to win gaining recognition for the effort. Sports may not be an option for other children, their achievements may be seen in mastering some of the tasks of everyday living. A hurdle is a hurdle no matter how big or small.

*   *   *

Hi! My name is Katie. I am a very special child with a disability, and there are some things that I cannot do. I cannot talk or write. But there are lots of things that I CAN do. What I do best is to have fun.

There have been times in my life when I have been in contests with sports. My mom is often my coach, and she works with me to learn how to do things right. Sometimes when I compete I do well and get a ribbon, a trophy, or a medal. I really like to show these to my family and friends.

One of the first times I competed was in a modified Special Olympics event in swimming. I was in a pool where the floor went up and down. This helped me when I wasn't a very strong swimmer yet. My mom was in the pool with me. I swam against three other swimmers. I don't remember how I did, but it got me started in competition.

Another time I remember is when I got my first baseball trophy. I was playing on a "Challenger" team with other kids with a disability. At the end of the season all of us received a baseball trophy. I was so excited that I kissed the trophy just like I had seen on TV! Everyone laughed, but I know that all those great athletes do that so I did too.

I have often had my picture in the paper for my skiing competitions. The Akron Beacon-Journal *has put my picture in their paper a few times when I am at Special Olympics Ohio Winter Games. I also was on the front page of the* Whitefish Pilot *when I was skiing in Montana. And I have been taped for TV a few times as well. It is great fun to replay these and to remember what I was doing. It reminds me of how much fun I have.*

Fifteen
Staying Active

Many Americans are overweight. The reasons for this are many and varied. The same reasons can affect the disabled. A mix of possible physical problems and a variety of deleterious genetic and metabolic factors compounds the possibility of weight gain. A child with mobility has an advantage in maintaining a healthy weight or losing excessive weight. Preventing excessive weight gain can be achieved by paying attention to diet and maintaining a healthy level of activity.

Daily walking is the simplest of exercises. The results benefit both the parent and the child. Your neighborhood is the obvious setting for this activity, but create interest by trying the zoo or a park or a trail. Walking on relatively level ground poses little or no threat to safe walking. Gradually increasing distance can strengthen legs, build muscles, and develop stamina—all components of a healthy individual.

Although it might be difficult to get your child to be active outside, we have found that a large three-wheel bike has been a great tool. When we first got the idea, we didn't know if Katie could even work the pedals or figure out how to make the bike stop. So we found an older used bike and fixed it up for her. We added a bell, a license plate with Katie's name, a huge orange flag, a new seat, and new handle grips with fringe on them. She loved it!

It was a bit of a struggle getting her to use the brakes. But she eventually understood the technique. The other problem was that our driveway is on a bit of a hill. At first, when returning home, she would ride to the base of the drive and get off and walk the bike up the slope of the driveway. Now she has mastered pushing the pedals and can come up and down the drive using her own power.

About a year ago we got her a new bike for her birthday. It was a huge success! We really were able to surprise her, and she truly loved the new bike. She has her own helmet, and I am sure she feels quite independent and free when she is out on the street. There are limits to how far she can ride, but we can usually see the orange flag, so we know where she is. It has been a wonderful tool and source of exercise.

*   *   *

Hi! My name is Katie. I am a very special child with a disability, and there are some things that I cannot do. I cannot talk or write. But there are lots of things that I CAN do. What I do best is have fun.

One of my favorite toys is my bike. It is lots bigger than the ones that my folks have and the one my brother had. But I can get around the neighborhood without having someone right with me all the time. That's fun.

Sometimes in the summer I ride the bike down to the neighborhood swim club and go for a swim. This is really nice because the parking lot sometimes is filled with cars. This way I can put my swim bag in my basket and lock my bike by the pool and not worry about where to find a parking place.

I also get to visit the neighbors when they are out in the lawn working. Everyone stops to say hi to me. And I stop for everyone. It is a great way to have fun.

Sixteen
Worship Stories

Whether a person ascribes to a religious belief or not is a deeply personal matter. At issue here are the benefits that can come from membership in a church community. Participation can provide a great source of comfort and a sense of belonging. It includes your child in yet another family structure. It provides a means of educating yet another group of people about those with disabilities.

As with all things, the benefits of a religious affiliation are dependent upon a level of commitment. You will get more out of active participation than simple membership. I have learned many valuable lessons at Church and been given some valuable advice from trusted friends. It is also a place of parental support.

If attending church has been a part of your normal family routine then continue and include your child with a disability if possible. Your family will relish holding on to a regular routine, and your child will enjoy being further incorporated into the family structure. As always, weigh the benefits of going to church with the level of your child's disabilities and the level of exposure you want your child to have.

Katie seems to enjoy the "spirituality" of the environment. She has watched and learned some of the protocol throughout the years. She also attended the rite of passage services that her brother was involved in. Eventually she participated in the same ceremonies. Her regular participation in the worship service is another way in which she feels valued and in which she feels she belongs.

Additionally, I believe her presence is a value to the community. We have been members of the same parish for twenty-five years. Many of our fellow parishioners have watched Katie grow up and have not only accepted her, but welcomed her participation. They share in her excitement over successes (Special Olympics) and comment on her cheerfulness.

Katie has truly been a blessing to our community. In fact, she often is more aware of the order of worship than much of the congregation. For starters, she knows all the responses, even though she cannot actually say them. She knows we begin our prayer with the Sign of the Cross, she knows when to sit and stand and kneel, and she tries to join in the "Alleluia" whenever it is sung. (She can sort of say her "l's.") If the presider sits in prayerful thought too long to suit her, she tries to stand up to move the service along. And if the choir leads us in too many verses of the recessional, she begins to get her coat on and move out of the pew. She definitely knows what is going on.

Two prime examples of this come to mind. The first event had to do with her reception of Catholic First Communion. In our faith tradition, when a person understands and believes in the sacredness of the reception of a Host and sip of wine, they are welcomed to receive the Eucharist, also called Holy Communion. This is assumed to be around the age seven or eight. Since we didn't know how she would react to the consumption of the Host and we were a little unsure of her particular theological level of understanding, we decided to have her receive the Eucharist for the first time at a very small weekday liturgy. There were probably only a dozen folks in attendance. She had practiced the proper procedure for the reception of the sacrament, and she did well. We were all a little misty-eyed, but it went beautifully. However, her real impression of the whole event emerged when we got ready to take her picture after the service. I tried to position her in front of the altar in the small chapel which was okay, but then she bolted and ran into the larger church to stand at the foot of the steps of the large sanctuary. I finally figured out that this is the spot where her brother had his picture taken and every other First Communion class that she had witnessed. She wanted her photo to be taken here as well. And so we did.

The second event came when she was confirmed some years later. She attended a class and worked on some projects with other students with disabilities. Her actual ceremony was to take place with the "regular" students, and she was to be the final one confirmed. The Bishop and I had discussed her possible inability to master the five steps to kneel at his feet, and he was going to rise from the Bishop's Chair and meet her at the bottom step. However, the end of the line came upon him rapidly, and he had not risen. No matter, Katie climbed up the steps to kneel at his feet as she had just witnessed some eighty others do. Her sponsor was hard pressed to keep up with her! It was quite a moment of triumph for Katie.

Many faith traditions have classes for youth instruction. Some have learning environments structured for those with a disability as well. If your faith community is really living their faith, then they should welcome you and your child each and every week. If they don't, find another faith community. There are plenty around.

Information can be found regarding religious opportunities for people with disabilities on the website for the National Organization on Disability, www.nod.org. Connect to the "Religion and Disability Program" which is an interfaith organization. This site also offers information on three guides published to assist families and to links to many other organizations.

*   *   *

Hi! My name is Katie. I am a child with a disability, and there are lots of things that I cannot do. I cannot read or write. But there are lots of things that I CAN do. I can ride a bike, and swim. But what I like to do best is to have fun.

I have been very blessed to grow up in a home where going to church was a part of every weekend. When I was little, my brother went with us all the time, and I really loved to sit with him and with my Mom. We had many friends who would sit near us, and I have come to know them over the years. In fact some of them will sit with us on purpose because they like me. My favorite part of the service is when we do the Sign of Peace. It is supposed to be a community time of shaking hands and well wishing. But in my area, it turns into a lot of hugging.

When I was very little I could not receive Communion. But I would usually walk up with my brother and Mom and receive a blessing. I wanted to receive Jesus in the Eucharist too, and Mom helped me to learn about it. I was very proud to receive the first time and every time. Mom keeps a close watch on me, and I do it right most of the time. But just about everyone knows me and understands if I don't get it right every time. It is great to see my friends at church. It is fun to go and give and receive many hugs.

Seventeen
Puppy Choice

The child with disabilities can have a great love of and interest in animals, and animals can give love and affection unconditionally. A match often made in heaven. Pets can be a great source of excitement and contentment for those with a disability. The animal does not make judgments and is usually available for loving on about any terms. But the family needs to be careful when choosing a household animal.

I know that various animal rescue and Humane Society programs often bring the "visiting dogs" to schools and workplaces. Animals are also residents at many nursing homes as a stable and loving presence. Katie loved the dog at my Mom's nursing home, and she loves the animal visits at her workplace.

We have always been able to keep a very calm and yet affirming pet in our house. By accident, we had a great pet when Katie was born, a yellow lab. Sparkle was a large female with a great love of children. She was calm, yet protective, easygoing, yet able to play forever. She was wonderful with kids in general, and Katie in particular.

When Sparkle died, we were fortunate enough to get a Golden Retriever who we named Flash. She was also a great choice. We bred her twice and exposed the kids to the birth process with two litters of puppies. It was a worthwhile experience, and Katie seemed to be totally in her element with the puppies. Much affection was exchanged.

We kept the firstborn of the second litter, Gipper, and he lived a long time. Now we have a black lab, Derby, and he is just as wonderful with Katie as the previous dogs. I think Katie feels safer with Derby in the house. He is very protective of her—the new bus driver had to go several weeks to be "approved." And all of the labs/retrievers are patient with Katie, don't seem to mind if she sits on them, and are continuously affectionate.

If there is an issue, it is that Katie assumes all pets are as openly caring as our dogs have been. Katie frequently tries to pet animals that belong to other people only to be rebuffed by a skittish small dog or a cat who has little use for people. Knowing about four-legged pets is a good area of training for Katie who is always a little too eager to meet and greet. We are constantly physically holding on to her when other dogs are around.

Choosing a pet should always be a family decision. Consider the nature of your child's disability and your own affinity for animals. The pet's needs must be considered as well. Families sometimes are constrained by the living conditions such as whether the yard is large enough or whether a park is nearby. Pets are great for children with disabilities. Choose wisely!!

*　　*　　*

Hi! My name is Katie. I am a special child with a disability, and there are some things that I cannot do. I cannot write or talk. But there are lots of things that I CAN do. I can swim, ride a bike, go skiing, and go just about everywhere. What I do best is to have fun.

One of the ways that I have fun is with my dog. I have lived in our house with four different dogs in my lifetime. I love dogs, especially the ones that I am around most of the time.

They let me lie on them and give them kisses and pull on their ears or tails. They have all been very good to me.

When I was little, we had two litters of puppies. I had no idea what was going on! It was neat to watch the puppies being born. And I got to help take care of them. They were also very good to me even though I often picked them up by their tails. If I sat on the lawn, all the puppies would jump on me and we would tumble around on the grass. I laughed a lot! But they all grew up and went to homes of our friends. Some of them we saw often and some we never saw again.

Also, we kept one of the puppies. What fun! Except I think he chewed on my shoes once, my new ones, and totally ruined them. Bad dog! But he grew up to be another fun member of the family, and he traveled with us everywhere.

Sometimes my parents worry about me, because I think all dogs are as nice and fun as my dogs. I have to be careful, because they all don't know me.

But if you ask me, get a lab! They're lots of fun!

Eighteen
Legal and $$$ Matters

Legal considerations and money matters are very closely related. How each is handled impacts the other. Laws and requirements regarding these issues vary from state to state. Having an attorney and social caseworker to guide you through these matters is crucial.

When Katie was very small, we were advised to rewrite our wills. This was done in order to establish a guardian for her in case of our deaths and to be sure NOT to leave her any money. The relationship goes like this:

1. Wills: The child with a disability must have very little or no money in order to qualify for some county, state and federal services, to receive benefits, and to stay "in the system." Once an income reaches a certain level, benefits could cease. Not good. Each county and state sets its own limit on income. We were advised to set up a "Bubble Gum" Trust that would be money used only for special purposes, beyond the daily needs.

2. Bank Account: The child will need a bank account into which the monthly government check can be deposited. This could be welfare or Social Security (SSI) or any other program for which she qualifies. The money cannot accumulate in this account! Ba-

sically this money must go to room and board, clothing, medical expenses, and entertainment. There is a semi-annual meeting with the county agency to account for all of this. The amount that is received will depend on family income, age of parents, and other factors. Federal programs should be the same across the country, but state and local agencies vary by region. It is important to get advice to keep you up to date as the laws and regulations as well as the agencies and programs are always changing.

3. Services: The services might include work opportunities, schooling, housing, food stamps, and waivers for care. There are probably additional services available, but these are the ones with which I am familiar. Again, the programs can vary by state and county. Application must be made with each agency in order for services to begin. It is wise to remain in one geographic location in order to maintain the services without having to reapply frequently.

4. Guardianship: When the child with a disability becomes an adult at age eighteen, a guardianship should be arranged. Again, this will go through the county court system and a yearly filing is required. The report contains information on any progress made by the individual, data on their living arrangements, and updates on medical information.

Learning all the requirements for each different service seemed to take forever. I still am nervous that I will fail to file something on time or spend too much money somewhere, or worse yet, not spend enough of her money. Katie lives at home, but there are many of her co-workers who live in group homes. In this case, I believe the housing agency takes care of all the paperwork and reports.

Legal and financial matters can be quite complex. Working with knowledgeable efficient caseworkers and attorneys can help ease the process. Most paperwork must be filed by certain dates. Make sure you are aware of these dates and write them in bold print on your calendar to avoid missing out on available benefits.

Nineteen
Special Education and Beyond

Education for the disabled has not always been available. Fortunately, laws were passed in the United States making it possible for all individuals with disabilities to receive an education. Since you will be the main advocate for your child, you should know about the laws that make education a civil right. Situations may develop where you may have to fight for your child's right to a fair education.

In 1975, the Education for All Handicapped Act (PL94–142) was passed. This law targeted individuals with disabilities, ages three to twenty-one, and provided for "free and appropriate education" in "the least restrictive environment." It also increased the rights of the parents to be involved in all educational decisions provided for the annual completion of an Individualized Education Plan (IEP). The IEP is a plan that is made by the parents, teachers, school administrators, and the student. It sets educational expectations for the coming year. This is a multi-paged, state document which is copied and distributed to everyone at the meeting. The IEP sets benchmarks for academic progress as well as physical, social, and behavioral expectations.

The Education for All Handicapped Act was amended in 1990 and was entitled the Individual with Disabilities Education Act (IDEA). The most important feature of this law was to require transition plans on every IEP by the age of sixteen.

This would help to chart the individual's course once formal schooling had ceased.

In 1997, amendments were made to IDEA ensuring access to the general education curriculum, strengthening the role of parents and guardians, and emphasizing student progress based on the IEP. It also set funding formulas.

All this legislation has been extremely helpful in providing an educational environment for children with disabilities and has been wonderful for Katie. In our area of the country, "grade levels" are in six-year increments, which give the student the opportunity to avoid disturbing yearly classroom transitions by allowing them to attend the same school, even remain in the same classroom with the same teacher, for six years. Because of this system, Katie was able to learn sign language and some basic socializing skills while in the same safe and stable surroundings, with the same teacher and same schools for six years.

As Katie aged, the next "class" was held in another school building with other students closer to her own age. In this environment the content of the academic curriculum included more practical skills such as counting, money usage, and vocational job skills.

Her final six years of education were in a regular high school building. One of the components of this program was to gain experience at a number of work facilities. Katie and her class trained at local hotels and motels learning housekeeping skills, at the Humane Society and various pet stores, and at local retail stores stocking shelves. These years helped teach us what she could accomplish and provided realistic goal-setting expectations for her future employers.

Upon graduation, Katie was employed. Although the opportunities for work are handled differently in every state and county, we found Katie fits best in a work environment that allows her to be fairly social yet sets expectations for her work load. Our area also provides transportation to and from work. Each bus has an aide to assist the driver each day. Katie loves taking the bus.

Work is a place to go to every day where Katie is with friends. It also enables her to bring home a small paycheck every few weeks. She loves going to work every day.

Twenty
Never Give Up

Never, ever give up. If you do, so will your child. You are their advocate for a lifetime. There will always be an agency or a school system that is willing to sacrifice your child's future to save a few bucks. If a program or a class or an activity is wrong for your child, you must speak out. Even in the face of daunting odds, never give up.

I had to learn and re-learn this lesson every summer. Katie was placed in a multi-handicapped class that was run by the county. This was because at her young age, the school system in our district offered no services. Our local district then was responsible for her transportation, even if it meant out-of-district bussing. Since they offered no alternative educational opportunity, they had to consent. This was fine until Katie was twelve years old.

When Katie turned twelve, the school district officials wanted to place her in a multi-handicapped class within the district rather than in the county class. I had researched this and found that the local class was not as good as the county class. The local class wasn't given the opportunity to pursue out of school job experiences, go on outings, and prepare for other life-skill options as was the county class. At Katie's IEP meeting, I would firmly establish that I wanted her to remain in the county program, regardless of the expenses incurred to the district due to transportation or fees. In May, they would agree. I would be assured that transportation would be arranged.

However, in July, I would find out that my wishes had been undermined by one of the school district officials, and that Katie was to be placed in the local class, not the county program. My anger was nearly uncontrollable. After numerous phone calls, much argument, and my own high blood pressure, Katie would be restored to the rolls of the county class. This happened for SIX years. Then it got worse.

When Katie turned eighteen, the county class was held in an adjoining district. The local school official, the assistant superintendent, refused to allow Katie to attend. Never mind that this is a parent's choice, she and her office refused to allow it. I sued them. I obtained free legal assistance from our state advocate organization, and I brought a lawsuit against them. The school district refused to back down. The state sent our lawyers to mediate. They refused. It was only hours before the court proceedings were to begin that the school district finally capitulated.

I have since found out that I am the only person in the history of our district to have won an argument with this particular district official and her office. Her goal was to save the district money; the welfare of the students, especially those most in need of attention, was of no concern. Parents of the disabled had been quite willing to defer to her and abdicate their parental right and responsibility. They gave up.

If you do not stand up for your child, for the future of your child, no one else will. Never, ever give up.

*   *   *

Hi! My name is Katie. I am a very special child with a disability, and there are some things that I cannot do. I cannot

talk or write. But there are lots of things that I CAN do. What I do best is have fun.

So many people have taught me things throughout my life. I have had some really great teachers who have been very helpful to me. They are my friends, and I will never forget them. It is great to see them when we are out shopping or at an event. They have helped me learn to have fun.

Now that I am older and I go to work every day, I still have fun. I still get to ride the yellow bus every day, and I still have some great drivers. And I have learned many new jobs at work, too. But we still do many other things besides work. We still get to go on field trips, and I have learned safety and dance at my work. So every day I still get to have fun.

Twenty-one
Keep Learning

Challenging yourself sets an example for your disabled child. Read. Investigate new programs. Examine the possibilities for new vacations. If you become complacent, so will your child.

If you are near a college or university, you have a great resource. Most of them have programs for teachers of those with a disability, or special education. They often have "clinics" for these prospective teachers. They are in need of pupils for these programs. Here is an opportunity for some inexpensive extra guidance for your child.

Katie has been involved with the speech program at the local university for about thirteen years. She registers each semester as our schedule allows. She loves it! There is a fee, but it is a whole new opportunity for her to work on skills with new clinicians who share their expertise. The student clinicians get to practice with Katie's communication board, a speaking device that has been programmed to speak for Katie, and then develop new ways for Katie to use it.

Some of the organizations for parents of those with disabilities are free. Watch your local newspaper for information on the times and locations of their meetings. A great deal can be learned about activities for both you and your child.

Publications for parents of those with special needs are available. Your local organizations for parents can inform you of these. Read them and find new ways to stimulate both your life and your child's life.

Get your child involved in Special Olympics and your county programs for the Special Needs child. They are active year-round with a multitude of sports activities. There are sports for each season, and volunteer coaches to assist in skill development. In addition, each state organization sponsors statewide competitions in nearly all of the athletics offered. This is another great opportunity for your child to learn new social skills, develop and use her athletic skills, and further develop a sense of value and independence.

There are literally hundreds of organizations that can be located in a web search. Try many of the various search engines. A search I conducted of "disability related organizations" yielded thirty-three organizations, with many of the organizations relating to specific types of disabilities such as blindness, deafness or spinal injury. Another search on Yahoo of Disability Organizations produced 120 sites further broken down into categories specializing in information on developmental disabilities or education or physical therapy. Other helpful sites were devoted to regional, state, and national groups.

*   *   *

Hi! My name is Katie. I am a special child with a disability, and there are some things that I cannot do. I cannot talk or write. But there are lots of things that I CAN do. What I do best is to have fun.

I go lots of places with my family. One of my favorite places to go is the county fair. There is so much to see and do there!

After we arrive, we usually walk up and down the midway. We have to see what the fair has to offer. We check out the rides, what kind of food they have, and where all the animals are.

After that, we decide which rides I will go on. This is great fun! I love to spin around and go up and down. Sometimes my folks ride with me, and sometimes they take pictures of me on the rides. Then I can look at them later.

Then I look at all the animals. There are so many! I like to touch them and see if their skin is soft. But I have to be careful. The horses are so tall, and the rabbits are so small. The roosters are so loud, and some of the animals are smelly.

Sometimes there is a competition for horsemanship. We sit in the stands and watch as the riders and horses go through the special skills. Sometimes I know some of the riders, and I cheer for them.

I usually get something to eat. Sometimes we eat an entire dinner, sometimes just a sandwich. And sometimes we eat ice cream or a candy apple.

The 4H clubs are also at the fair. They show off all of their work and all of the things that they make. Sometimes they are working on projects while we are there.

I really like to go the fair at night. The rides all run with their lights on. The Ferris wheel looks so pretty way up in the sky.

There are lots of things to see and do at the county fair and all of them are fun!

Twenty-two
Encourage Independence

Encourage your child to be independent. Performing most tasks on your own will probably be quicker and easier in the short term, but your child can most probably learn to be successful in many ways. Remember to temper your expectations, because the timetable for these accomplishments will not fit a "normal" schedule. Just remember to never give up. You will be surprised at what you and your child can learn!

Begin with toileting skills. This will allow you more independence as well! Develop a routine; set routine times. Make the experience positive and not fearful. Be a gentle guide. Helpful in this endeavor is the type of clothing that you have chosen. Your child should be wearing pants with elastic, shirts that pull on, and shoes that have Velcro closings. In the summer, sandals are a good bet. Use a jacket that has a zipper instead of buttons. The confidence that this will give your child will be rewarded with new attempts at independence.

Perhaps your child can learn some kitchen skills. Setting the table is a fairly safe project. You can make a plastic placemat that has drawings of "what goes where" until the pattern is learned. Then clearing the table after a meal becomes less frightening. Also plastic makes emptying of the dishwasher less of a threat. Eventually, your child may be able to get their own drink, make a sandwich, even if all they are doing in the beginning is watching you and making their own choices.

Establishing a bedtime routine also helps foster independence. Set bath time at a predictable schedule, and then perhaps allow your child to actually go to bed when they are tired.

It also helps if along the way you allow your child some independence in choices concerning clothes to wear, places to go, towels to use, and the like. Their independence is also a small step towards your independence.

*   *   *

Hi! My name is Katie. I am a special child with a disability, and there are some things that I cannot do. I cannot talk or write. But there are lots of things that I CAN do. What I do best is have fun.

I have been able to do some dressing of myself for a while now, and it is a fun thing to be able to do. When I was very young, my Mom dressed me all the time and took my clothes off for my bath.

But I began to learn how to undress myself first. It was lots of fun to have all my clothes off before Mom even got in the bathroom to start the bath! It was also fun to get my clothes off to be ready to get my swim suit on.

It has taken longer for me to learn how to put clothes on. I began with socks and shoes. Sometimes I still put my shoes on the wrong feet, but I can get them on.

If my clothes are laid out for me, I can get on my shirt and my pants. I don't always know the back from the front, but I am learning about labels. A trick that my Mom uses is to put my name on the back of my underpants so I know where the back is, and then I know how to put them on.

When I see the bus coming or know we are going out, it is nice to know that I can dress myself. It makes it a little more fun for me and for Mom.

Twenty-three
Balance

This is my motto. Please put it on my tombstone. *Balance your life with the life of your child.* I have come to realize that I can never schedule anything for myself without first accounting for Katie. Yes, it is difficult. But it must be done. For your own health and well-being, you have to balance activities. You need to learn to balance learning with fighting for the rights of your child. You may have to adjust your own immediate goals to make accommodations for your child, but be sure to return to them when the time allows.

As your disabled child grows, learns, achieves, and perhaps, becomes independent, you will not have forgotten who you are and what is important. You will create many happy memories and have risen to that most noble challenge of all—to be a parent.

Conclusion

Although this appears to be the end of my "hot tips" on helping a child with a disability to grow into a young adult, I am sure it will not be the end of my learning or my family's experiences. Every day we learn new things that Katie can do, and we need to make our own adjustments. Her learning continues as well. I know that she is not "done" yet; therefore, neither are we.

The challenge of passing these skills on to Katie's brother continues. The probability exists that he will teach Katie some new skills too. Maybe one day there will be another book, only that one will be titled, *I'm Katie's Brother.*